Dealing with Alcoholic Hepatitis:

A Personal Relief Code for the disease

Written by

Fernando A. Larrison

Table of Contents

Introduction

The purpose of this book is to increase awareness of the frequently ignored and underappreciated ailment known as alcoholic hepatitis. We want to provide a thorough explanation of this liver illness, including its causes, diagnosis, therapy, and prospective, by delving deeply into its complexity.

Alcohol abuse can result in alcoholic hepatitis, a kind of liver inflammation. It is a cunning foe that frequently emerges covertly in those who consume alcohol heavily or repeatedly. Despite being stealth, alcoholic hepatitis can cause serious liver damage and even life-threatening complications if undiagnosed and untreated.

We set out on a voyage through the pages of this book to understand the underlying causes of alcoholic hepatitis and investigate the clinical presentation and diagnostic equipment. We will look into pharmaccutical therapies, dietary support, and lifestyle changes as part of the medical management of alcoholic hepatitis. We'll also talk about sophisticated treatment alternatives like liver transplantation and the challenges of managing consequences.

In addition, we explore prevention, emphasizing the value of public health programs, and alcohol awareness campaigns in reducing the effects of alcoholic hepatitis. Early detection and treatment by medical professionals are crucial to halting the spread of this disease and improving patient outcomes.

It's crucial to remember that this book cannot replace specific medical advice or clinical consultation. The information presented here is meant to be a resource that will help readers learn more about alcoholic hepatitis. The services of qualified healthcare specialists should be sought out for customized diagnosis, treatment, and management programs.

We anticipate that "Exposing the Covert Enemy: Understanding Alcoholic Hepatitis" will be a useful tool for researchers, doctors, patients, and their families. We hope to have a substantial influence on the lives of those who are impacted by alcoholic hepatitis by raising awareness, enhancing diagnosis, and developing treatment approaches.

Alcoholic Hepatitis: An outline

Alcohol consumption results in alcoholic hepatitis, which is liver inflammation. It can also be seen as a state of escalating inflammatory liver damage brought on by chronic excessive ethanol consumption.

People who drink heavily over a long period of time have a higher risk of developing alcoholic hepatitis. Over a ten-year period, alcohol use above 20 g/day for women and 60 g/day for males greatly increases the relative chance of developing cirrhosis. Alcoholic hepatitis and drinking, however, have a complicated association. Alcoholic hepatitis can strike even moderate drinkers, and it doesn't always affect heavy drinkers.

If severe drinking continues, alcoholic hepatitis usually persists and develops into cirrhosis. If drinking stops, alcoholic hepatitis gradually goes away over a period of weeks to months, perhaps with no long-term effects but frequently with lingering cirrhosis.

You must stop drinking if you have been told that you have alcoholic hepatitis. A high risk of fatal liver disease and death exists for those who continue to consume alcohol.

Signs and Symptoms

For an early diagnosis and prompt treatment, it's essential to be aware of the signs and symptoms of alcoholic hepatitis. Here are some typical warning signs and symptoms of this condition:

- Abdominal Pain: People with alcoholic hepatitis frequently feel uneasy or painful in the upper right corner of the belly. This discomfort can range in severity and be either dull or acute.
- Jaundice: A common sign of liver malfunction is yellowing of the skin and eyes, also known as jaundice.

Jaundice develops in alcoholic hepatitis as a result of the liver's decreased capacity to handle bilirubin.

- Weariness and Weakness: People with alcoholic hepatitis frequently complain of chronic weariness and weakness. These symptoms can have a crippling effect on daily tasks.

- Loss of Appetite: Alcoholic hepatitis can cause appetite loss, which might unintentionally cause weight loss. Nutritional deficits may make the illness worse.

- Vomiting and persistent nausea: This are two symptoms that some people with alcoholic hepatitis encounter. These signs and symptoms may be related to electrolyte imbalances and dehydration.

- Spider angiomas: On the surface of the skin, spider angiomas appear as tiny, red, spider-like blood vessels. People with alcoholic liver disease are more likely to experience them.

- Swelling and Fluid Retention: Alcoholic hepatitis can lead to fluid buildup in the abdomen, which can cause swelling or abdominal distention. Due to fluid retention, swollen ankles or legs may also be seen.

- Mental Disorientation: Alcoholic hepatitis can, in extreme cases, result in hepatic encephalopathy, a disorder that is marked by mental disorientation, memory issues, and behavioral disturbances.

The intensity of symptoms might vary, and it is crucial to remember that not everyone with alcoholic hepatitis will suffer the same ones. Furthermore, because these symptoms and signs might coexist with those of other liver diseases, a precise diagnosis is essential.

It is crucial to consult a doctor for an accurate evaluation, diagnosis, and treatment if you or someone you know exhibits any of these symptoms and has a history of binge drinking. The problem can be managed and additional liver damage can be avoided with prompt management.

Risk factors and causes of alcoholic hepatitis

Heavy drinking over a lengthy period of time is the primary cause of alcoholic hepatitis. Alcohol metabolism in the liver results in inflammation that may kill liver cells.

As time passes, the body's functional liver tissue is gradually replaced by scars. The liver's functionality is hampered by this.

Causes

The last stage of alcoholic liver disease is irreversible scarring, sometimes known as cirrhosis.

As the condition worsens, cirrhosis can quickly lead to liver failure. The blood supply to the kidneys may also be hampered by a diseased liver. Damage and renal failure could be the results of this.

Alcoholic hepatitis can also be caused by other reasons, such as:

- More hepatitis varieties: You are more prone to develop cirrhosis if you have hepatitis C and also consume alcohol, even in moderation.

- Malnutrition: Because they eat poorly or because alcohol and its metabolites inhibit the body from adequately absorbing nutrients, many heavy drinkers are undernourished. Damage to liver cells is a result of nutritional deficiencies.

Risk factors

Your alcohol consumption is the main risk factor for developing alcoholic hepatitis. It is unknown how much alcohol is necessary to increase your chance of contracting alcoholic hepatitis. However, the majority of those who have the illness have a history of drinking more than 3.5 ounces (100 grams) every day for at least 20 years, which is equal to seven glasses of wine, seven beers, or seven shots of booze.

However, even those who don't drink as much and have other risk factors can get alcoholic hepatitis.

Other danger signs consist of:

- Sex: Because women digest alcohol differently than men, they appear to be at a higher risk of getting alcoholic hepatitis.

- Obesity: Alcoholic hepatitis and the progression from that illness to cirrhosis may be more likely to develop in heavy drinkers who are overweight.

- genetic influences: Although it can be challenging to distinguish between genetic and environmental influences, studies have suggested that alcohol-induced liver damage may have a hereditary component.

- A drinking binge: For men, having five or more drinks within two hours, and for women, having four or more, may raise your risk of developing alcoholic hepatitis.

- Racial and ethnic background: Alcoholic hepatitis may be more common in Blacks and Hispanics.

Disease Development: Genetic and Environmental Aspects

Genetic and environmental factors work together to determine the onset of alcoholic hepatitis. Understanding how these elements interact will help us better understand the risk factors and underlying causes of the disease. In this article, we examine the genetic and environmental factors that may contribute to the onset of alcoholic hepatitis:

Genetic influences:

- Genetic Predisposition: A person's vulnerability to alcohol-related liver illnesses, such as alcoholic hepatitis, can be increased by specific genetic variants. The onset of liver injury may be influenced by variations in genes related to alcohol metabolism, inflammation, and antioxidant pathways.

- Family history: A genetic susceptibility to developing alcoholic hepatitis can be revealed by a family history of alcoholic liver illnesses. People who have close relatives who have had liver problems brought on by alcohol may be at a higher risk of getting the ailment themselves.

Environmental Factors:

- Consumption of Alcohol: Alcohol abuse is the primary epidemiological risk factor for hepatitis. Due to social, cultural, and religious variables, alcohol consumption varies greatly by location, with the highest amounts occurring in Europe and the United States and the lowest in South-East Asia and the nations of the eastern Mediterranean. As a result, alcohol-related ailments are more common in developed countries. There is a dose-dependent increase in the risk of hepatitis in those who use a lot of alcohol (40 g/day for women and 60 g/day for males), according to a number of sizable prospective cohort studies. According to a population survey, people who use more than 30 grams of alcohol each day are more likely to experience hepatitis and alcoholic liver damage.

- Malnutrition: In those who drink alcohol, liver damage can become worse due to poor nutrition, especially when diets are lacking in important vitamins and minerals. A person's susceptibility to alcoholic hepatitis increases when malnutrition impairs the liver's capacity to heal and rejuvenate.

- Coexisting Liver Diseases: Regardless of a lesser amount of alcohol intake, the possibility of developing alcoholic hepatitis can rise in people with a history of other liver disorders such non-alcoholic fatty liver disease (NAFLD) or viral hepatitis.

It is complicated and individualized how genetic and environmental variables interact. While some people may have a higher tolerance owing to genetic reasons but are still at danger when ingesting excessive amounts of alcohol, other people may develop alcoholic hepatitis even when they consume moderate amounts of alcohol.

Healthcare practitioners can more accurately determine a person's risk, offer suitable counseling, and create tailored interventions to prevent and manage alcoholic hepatitis by acknowledging the importance of hereditary and environmental factors. Future identification of genetic markers and the development of specific approaches to both treatment and prevention are also encouraged by continuing research in genomics and personalized medicine.

Tools for Diagnosis of Alcoholic Hepatitis

In order to accurately diagnose alcoholic hepatitis, a variety of instruments and tests must be used to examine liver function, gauge the severity of liver damage, and distinguish it from other liver disorders. The following are important tools frequently used in the diagnosis of alcoholic hepatitis:

History and Examination

Establishing if the patient abuses alcohol is a key clinical factor in the diagnosis of alcoholic Hepatitis. Nevertheless, making this choice is not always simple.

Alcohol usage is frequently downplayed or covered up by alcoholic patients and even their family members. To determine the true degree of alcohol usage, it is frequently essential to question a number of family members. Because of the relationship between the patient and caregiver, the level of trust, the method and tenacity caregivers may employ while acquiring the alcohol history, different carers frequently obtain divergent histories from the patient.

A medical examination can indicate symptoms including ascites (abdominal fluid buildup), ascites, abdominal discomfort, and enlarged liver.

Hepatic Biopsies and Histology

Alcoholic hepatitis is frequently diagnosed based on clinical and laboratory symptoms, but some diagnostic uncertainty may still exist in the absence of histological confirmation. This is due to improvements in serologic and genetic diagnosis of infectious and metabolic hepatitides over the past ten years.

Liver biopsy is frequently helpful to confirm the diagnosis and assess the severity of liver damage, however patients who have coagulopathy and/or thrombocytopenia run the risk of complications from this surgery. As a result, different skilled clinical hepatologists will employ liver biopsy in these patients, and the risk-benefit ratio of the procedure must be tailored in the clinical environment based on the desired level of diagnostic certainty.

Laboratory tests and Imaging studies While some laboratory abnormalities can be used for prognosis and represent the severity of alcohol-induced liver damage, others are simply helpful for diagnosis. Absent concurrent acetaminophen misuse, transaminase values are raised less than 5 to 10 times the usual amount. A reverse in this ratio indicates the presence of concurrent viral hepatitis or, alternatively, non-alcoholic steatohepatitis since the Aspartate Transferase (AST) level is nearly always higher than the alanine aminotransferase (ALT) level.

Acute viral hepatitis and alcoholic hepatitis can be distinguished from one another by looking at both the low rate of growth and the preponderance of the AST level. The predictive value of transaminase levels is ineffective, nevertheless. In more moderate to severe alcoholic hepatitis, prothrombin time and bilirubin levels are also raised, and the presence of leukocytosis and distress in the right upper abdomen quadrant may suggest biliary system disease.

Scoring Methods

The Glasgow Alcoholic Hepatitis Score (GAHS), the Model for End-Stage Liver Disease (MELD), and other scoring systems are used to evaluate the severity of alcoholic hepatitis and forecast its prognosis.

These diagnostic resources help establish a precise diagnosis of alcoholic hepatitis and direct effective treatment approaches when combined and interpreted by healthcare professionals. For an accurate assessment, a specific treatment plan, and the interpretation of test results, it is crucial to speak with trained medical specialists.

Prevention of Alcoholic Hepatitis

The main goals of preventing alcoholic hepatitis are to cut back on or stop drinking alcohol and to take care of the risk factors that go along with it. People can drastically lower their risk of contracting alcoholic hepatitis by taking preventive steps. The following are crucial tactics for preventing alcoholic hepatitis:

Alcohol Abstinence:

The best defense against alcoholic hepatitis is full abstinence from alcohol. This holds true for both those who have never consumed alcohol and those who have abused alcohol in the past.

If you currently drink, getting expert assistance, such as via counseling or support groups, can help you achieve and maintain abstinence.

Healthy Life Style and Nutrition:

A healthy lifestyle must be maintained if alcoholic hepatitis is to be avoided. Maintain a healthy weight, eat a balanced diet full of fruits, vegetables, and whole grains, and get frequent exercise.

A healthy diet is crucial since it promotes liver wellness and lowers the chance of inflammation brought on by alcohol. By eating a diet that is well-balanced or by taking supplements, be sure that you are getting enough of the critical vitamins and minerals.

Intervention and Support Mechanisms:

For those who struggle with alcohol misuse, creating support networks and seeking professional help are essential. Reaching out to medical professionals, addiction specialists, or support groups can offer advice, assistance and tools for prevention and treatment if you or someone you love has trouble managing alcohol usage.

The main focus of preventing alcoholic hepatitis is encouraging sensible alcohol use and adopting educated lifestyle decisions. People can lower their chance of getting alcoholic hepatitis and safeguard the health of their livers by putting abstinence, moderation, and healthy living first. Never forget that it is never too late to make positive changes or ask for assistance.

Treating the Covert Enemy

Avoiding consuming alcohol is the main therapeutic option for alcoholic hepatitis. Abstinence from alcohol may help repair liver damage in cases of early diagnosis. It can nevertheless aid in halting the progression of the illness in more severe cases.

Patients can explore options like therapy, medication, and detoxification programs with their doctor to safely reduce their alcohol usage.

Alcoholic hepatitis currently has no known cure, however treatment will work to lessen or eliminate symptoms and halt the disease's progression. Although the liver may partially restore the damage, liver scarring is a permanent condition.

The aim of treatment is to get the liver as close to normal as feasible. Some possibilities include:

Changing your diet Nutritional support:

A doctor could advise doing so. If a person is malnourished as a result of frequent alcohol usage, vitamin supplements or a targeted diet plan may assist to restore the body's nutritional balance.

A typical diet with 100 g/d of protein is suitable for persons with moderate alcoholic hepatitis. Offer additional folate and thiamine as well as multivitamins and minerals. Patients with ascites may need to limit their salt intake.

Medication:

To assist lessen liver inflammation, doctors may give drugs such as corticosteroids and pentoxifylline.

For patients who have achieved abstinence, naltrexone or acamprosate may be given in conjunction with psychotherapy to help them prevent relapsing. Although prednisolone and pentoxifylline are advised for the treatment of severe alcoholic hepatitis, their effectiveness is still debatable.

Transplantation of the liver:

Patients with advanced liver disease frequently receive orthotopic liver transplants. Due to persistent alcohol misuse, the majority of individuals with active alcoholic hepatitis are ineligible for transplantation. Prior to being evaluated for a liver transplant in the majority of American liver transplant programs, patients must abstain from alcohol for at least six months, and a complete psychosocial assessment must show that patients have a low likelihood of returning to alcohol misuse.

Patients with alcoholic hepatitis may be told that after abstaining from alcohol for at least six months, their liver damage should lessen and their liver function should improve. If they stay dedicated to continuous abstinence, they may be eligible for transplantation if they nonetheless develop cirrhosis and its consequences. The possibility of a liver transplant can be a strong motivator to promote abstinence.

Consultations:

Most cases of mild and severe alcoholic hepatitis can be treated on the medical floor of a hospital, necessitating just a short hospital stay. In fact, those who have the mostmild forms of the illness might never seek medical attention or might be successfully managed in an outpatient setting. However, severe acute alcoholic hepatitis necessitates multidisciplinary treatment and intense medical attention.

Extended Monitoring:

Patients can typically be discharged from severe medical rehabilitation establishments once signs of dependency on alcohol have subsided, the patient's liver condition has begun to improve, and issues from hepatic failure have begun to emerge. This is assuming there are no further issues.

Moving patients with a possibility for rehabilitation to an intensive drug misuse treatment program rather than releasing them from the hospital may be the best course of action.

In general, patients who have just been released from the hospital after experiencing an acute case of alcoholic hepatitis should be checked out within two weeks of their release. Following therapy, patients should have periodic follow-up appointments every few weeks to several months to assess their progress, check their electrolyte levels, get the results of a liver test, and support their recovery.

Remember that for individualized care and long-term maintenance, prompt intervention is critical, as is obtaining medical guidance and assistance. The secret adversary of alcoholic hepatitis can be confronted head-on with a comprehensive strategy, improving results and giving those affected new hope.

Research Advances and Promising Directions

Research breakthroughs are deepening our knowledge of alcoholic hepatitis and opening the door for novel methods to treatment, diagnosis, and prevention. Scientists and medical professionals are currently looking at novel approaches to enhance results and revolutionize the treatment of alcoholic hepatitis. Here are some recent research developments and promising field directions:

Predictors and Biomarkers:

Novel biomarkers are being investigated by researchers as a way to track treatment efficacy, identify those at risk of developing alcoholic hepatitis, and forecast the course of the disease. These biomarkers may help with individualized therapy choices and offer useful insights into the disease's underlying causes.

There is potential for enhanced risk categorization, prognosis assessment, and treatment planning with the creation of prediction models employing a combination of clinical, laboratory, and genetic data.

Specialized Treatments:

Researchers are looking towards tailored treatments that target particular biological processes and mechanisms associated with alcoholic hepatitis. These treatments have the capacity to lessen liver inflammation, encourage regeneration, and stop the spread of the illness.

The effectiveness of antioxidants, anti-inflammatory pharmaceuticals, and immune-modulating treatments in lowering liver damage and improving outcomes in people with alcoholic hepatitis is being studied.

Personalized Medicine:

Research on alcoholic hepatitis is increasingly embracing the idea of personalized medicine, which involves treating each patient according to their particular characteristics. Healthcare providers can create tailored treatment plans based on a patient's genetic profile, disease severity, and response to treatment.

Individualized interventions and tailored medicines may be developed as a result of advances in genomics and the discovery of particular genetic markers linked to alcoholic hepatitis.

Gut-Liver Axis:

In the field of alcoholic hepatitis, there is now significant study on the complex interaction between the gut microbiome and liver health. The relationship between the gut and liver can be studied to learn how dysbiosis (imbalances in gut bacteria) affects liver inflammation and to find possible therapeutic targets.

Probiotics and other methods are being investigated as ways to modify the gut microbiota and enhance liver function in alcoholic hepatitis.

Clinical Trials and Joint Initiatives:

Modern clinical trials are assessing the effectiveness and security of novel therapeutic approaches for the treatment of alcoholic hepatitis. Individuals have the chance to receive cutting-edge treatments and advance medical knowledge by taking part in clinical trials.

To address the problems associated with alcoholic hepatitis, researchers, medical professionals, and patient advocacy organizations are working together to enhance knowledge sharing, data sharing, and multidisciplinary methods.

We hope to improve alcoholic hepatitis early identification, improve treatment effectiveness, and finally stop the disease from progressing by embracing these research advancements and promising prospects. The care of alcoholic hepatitis has a lot of room for improvement, and more study and collaboration could change it, giving those who have this difficult liver condition fresh hope.

Conclusion

In summary, alcoholic hepatitis is a significant liver disease that necessitates multifaceted methods to diagnosis, prevention, and therapy. We can avert the onset of alcoholic hepatitis and the difficulties that go along with it by emphasizing the value of abstaining from alcohol, encouraging safe drinking habits, and taking care of hereditary and environmental issues.

We can precisely detect alcoholic hepatitis and gauge its severity by early diagnosis, using diagnostic methods such medical history, physical examination, laboratory tests, imaging techniques, and liver biopsy. This makes it possible for medical experts to create individualized treatment regimens that put an emphasis on nutritional assistance, pharmaceutical therapies, managing problems, and stopping drinking.

As time goes on, it is critical to keep spreading awareness, educate people about the dangers of alcohol abuse, and offering support networks to encourage abstinence or moderate alcohol usage. Collaboration among medical professionals, researchers, patients, and their support systems can significantly improve alcoholic hepatitis prevention, detection, and management.

Let's work toward a time when the effects of alcoholic hepatitis are reduced, new therapies are developed as a result of research advances, and those who are impacted by this ailment can have happier, healthier lives. Together, we can overcome the difficulties caused by alcoholic hepatitis and build a future that is better for everyone.

Dealing with Alcoholic Hepatitis

www.ingramcontent.com/pod-product-compliance
Lightning Source LLC
Chambersburg PA
CBHW071117260726
48661CB00006B/2631